The writing process:
how to write a scientific article in one day

Jacob Rosenberg, MD, DSc, FACS

Copyright © 2019 by Jacob Rosenberg

All rights reserved.

No part of this book may be reproduced, distributed, or transmitted in any form or by any means, including photocopying, recording, or other electronic or mechanical methods, without the prior written permission of the author, except in the case of brief quotations embodied in articles or reviews.

ISBN: 9781693201448

The writing process: how to write a scientific article in one day

ULTIMATE RESEARCHER'S GUIDE SERIES
VOLUME 4

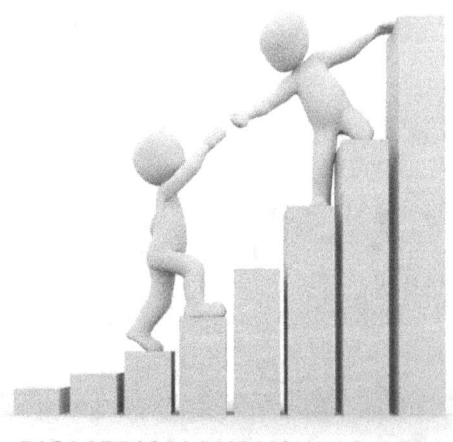

Table of contents

Preface 1

Chapter 1: Introduction to optimized writing habits 3
    Introduction 4
    How to overcome writer's block 9
    Criteria for evaluation of papers by journals 21

Chapter 2: Things to consider 28
    Composition of an original article 29
    Other article types 44
    Criteria for authorship 52
    Reference management software 56
    Problems with internet references 61

Chapter 3: Manuscript-map 64
    General preparations 65
    Manuscript mapping 73
    Exercise 85

Chapter 4: Prepare for dictation 86
    Required equipment 87
    How to prepare equipment and software
        95
    Exercise 102

Chapter 5: Dictation and revision of first draft
        103
    Dictation 104
    Revision of the first draft 109

Chapter 6: A few style tips 116
    Clear paragraph typography 117
    Delete unnecessary text 119
    Avoid certain terms and fillers 124
    Avoid name dropping 128
    Medical writing tips and tricks 130

Chapter 7: Closing 152
    closing remarks 153
    Other books in this series 155
    About the author 158
    Notes 159
    Contact information 161

Preface

This is the fourth book in a series where I will guide you through the different parts of the scientific process in order to improve the overall quality of your research project and thereby hopefully making it easier for you to get your scientific article published in a biomedical journal. We have now reached the phase where you should write your scientific paper based on your research results.

We have developed an effective method for speedy scientific writing where you prepare systematically for the writing process, and then dictate the manuscript to a smartphone. The sound file is then transcribed automatically, and with this technique you will most likely overcome "writer's block". The present book is called "The writing process: how to write a scientific article in one day" and it will guide you through the writing process and teach you the most effective way to overcome writer's block. In this way you will actually get it done and not sit and stare at the computer screen for hours without typing anything.

This special technique involves a preparation phase where you develop a manuscript map but without writing full sentences. Thereafter, you are able to dictate your entire scientific paper in one single day using a smartphone. In fact, the technique is so effective that you can dictate a full PhD thesis in a single day!

I have used this technique for many years and also taught it to several colleagues with great success. In my research unit all the researchers use it, and with this effective techniques they are each able to produce three scientific papers per year. I therefore hope, that you will find it interesting and will try it yourself. I can assure you that it is effective and it kills writer's block.

Enjoy!

Chapter 1: Introduction to optimized writing habits

Introduction

There is no doubt that there is pressure for a biomedical researcher to publish scientific articles. In the beginning of your career it matters more that you publish a number of papers rather than the quality of the papers themselves. This may sound strange but when you send an application for a new job or for research funding and you don't have many years of experience, then it is typical for the evaluators to look at your publication list.

    A new researcher will of course not be able to publish papers on the ultimate cure for cancer in the beginning of the career. You have to crawl before you can walk, so typically the first papers you will publish are not ground-breaking scientific news. This also makes sense from an educational point of view because performing research and writing scientific articles is a craft that has to be learned. Therefore, it is natural to publish less important and less difficult paper in the beginning of the career, and later, when you have become an expert in your field, then the scientific value of the papers will most typically increase. Thus, the quality of your research will evolve with time and experience. However, it does not in any way mean that technical quality of the scientific paper will increase with experience. You can easily write (dictate) papers of high technical quality if you use a reproducible and easy driving map for the process, and this is what I will teach you.

What matters?

- **Only your list of publications matters**
- **It doesn't matter if you were the coffee-master or a party-girl**
- **If you were research fellow for a year and only published one paper it actually gives a negative impression**

When you have had a period with fulltime research it does not matter afterwards if you were the coffee master or the party girl of your research group. The only thing that actually matters after your dedicated research period is the number of publications on your publication list. Of course the quality of the research also matters but to be honest, the number of papers is of great importance especially in the beginning of your career. It is therefore wise to focus on production of scientific articles in the first years of your research career.

Writer's block

Why don't you publish more?

- Fear of rejection and critique
- Lack of formal structure
- Lack of understanding of the editorial process
- Fear of suboptimal language
- Lack of time

In this context it is often a big problem that many first-time authors (and even older colleagues) will experience writer's block when they try to compose a scientific article. This is the main reason behind this book because you will be introduced to a new technique for scientific writing where writer's block will be eliminated or at least greatly reduced.

The trick is actually not rocket science, but you have to follow a certain work plan in order to obtain your goal and the goal is to write a full scientific article in only one day!

Why this book ?

- **Special concept**
  - **Manuscript mapping (outline)**
  - **Mind-to-paper (dictation)**

- **No-one else can write a paper (or a thesis...) in one day**

This special concept involves something called "manuscript mapping", where the scientific article is outlined in detail before the writing process actually starts. Then the actual writing process is not by typing on a computer, but instead you will need a smartphone to dictate the full manuscript of your article except for a few sections (see later in this book). To the best of my knowledge no one else can write a paper or even a full PhD-thesis in only one day and you will be able to do that when you have read this book and follow the instructions for this special concept of scientific writing.

How to overcome writer's block

Now we will discuss a very common and very irritating phenomenon. Writer's block means that you cannot get started – you can perhaps recognize the situation where you are sitting with your computer, fingers on the keyboard and then nothing happens. You try to write something, you are looking at the blinking curser on the screen and nothing happens. I guess all researchers have experienced writer's block somewhere in their career. It is not a phenomenon only for the young and inexperienced and even many older professors can tell you that they experience writer's block quite often. Writer's block is a well-known and heavily studied phenomenon in the pedagogic literature and there are several possible reasons for authors to experience writer's block.

Writer's block is the phenomenan that you may experience when you sit down to type text on your computer and then instead of typing you stop and go to get a cup of coffee or check your e-mails or facebook account and so on. These are all symptoms of writer's block and they will impair the writing process. This is extremely irritating and you have to find ways of getting around this.

It may be caused by different factors. Probably, and most importantly, it is caused by a fear of not doing the best you can. Fear of not writing good enough, you may have fear of rejection and fear of criticism and this is of course nonsense. However, we are all humans, so we may lack some self-confidence and this may be an important factor behind writer's block.

Another reason could be the lack of a formal structure of what you are about to write, and this can be tackled by better preparation. Writer's block may also be caused by a lack of understanding of the publication process. Few actually know what is happening at the editorial office and what factors will determine if the paper will be accepted or rejected.

There may also be some uncertainty about what level of language that you should use in a scientific paper, and I am a strong advocate for writing in simple English. Don't use very sophisticated terminology because nobody can read this, nobody can understand it and for you as an author or writer of scientific papers it is actually also quite difficult. If you have fear of suboptimal language I can assure you that this fear is stupid. You actually need to use suboptimal language in the sense that the language should not be overly complicated and that is one of the main reasons also to dictate your article instead in writing it yourself. It is important to use easy readable language which will give the reader a high speed of reading without stopping and having to read sentences all over again in over to simply understand what you are saying. So don't be afraid of using suboptimal language. Your spoken English is most probably of high enough quality that you can dictate your fist article draft and then later revise it to reach a format that can be submitted to a scientific journal. And don't use too difficult language because it will also be a contributing factor for your writer's block.

Another issue could be lack of time because if you feel stressed on time, then you may also perform worse. Therefore, prepare sufficiently, set enough time aside for the writing process and then perhaps you can avoid at least some of the writer's block. The best advice is probably to split the work for producing your article into different phases. The preparation phase can be performed during maybe a few months' time and you don't have to allocate full days for this. In this preparation phase you will develop your detailed outline, the manuscript map and prepare the dictation of the paper. When you dictate in your full first draft of the article you have to allocate enough time to do that in one single session. This is because during the dictation of the article you have to be quite concentrated and the dictation of a typical original article will probably take about 3-4 hours of concentrated work. You only use your references during this concentrated dictation time and afterwards in the revision phase, you can spend time on your manuscript also if you only have short periods available, maybe an hour here and there. The concentrated brain work is actually in the dictation phase, and this is why you have to allocate enough time for this to produce your first full article draft in one single session.

Overcoming writer's block

- **Getting started is the hardest part**

- **No shame in resorting to crutches**
  - Dictaphone
  - Modular writing - start with what is at the top of your mind

When you want to overcome writer's block it is probably the hardest part to get started. In order to do that it is strongly advisable to dictate the article instead of writing it yourself. Somehow, most people don't have difficulties speaking where they may experience writer's block when they have to type the text themselves on a PC keyboard. This is why it is an extremely good idea to dictate your paper instead of writing it yourself. Years ago we used dictaphones with tapes that were later transcribed verbatim by a secretary or by you. Nowadays it is much easier done by using a smartphone where you will produce a digital sound-file that can later be transcribed automatically by voice recognition software.

If you are not a talker by nature and you want to write yourself then you can do something else. You can use so-called modular writing. This means that you start with what is at the top of your mind, meaning what would you most like to write. Very often in an original paper the easiest part of the paper to write would be the title page. That is very easy to start with – and then the method section. The method section is straight forward. This is what has been written in your research protocol. It is a good idea to start with the title page and the method section and then you have started the process and will probably get a better writing flow to go to the other sections of the paper. This is called modular writing.

Overcoming writer's block

- **Find an environment with no distractions**
  - Long drives
  - Walking around
  - Borrowed beach house or motel room

- **Eliminate distractions in common environment**
  - Hard to control this one

Another trick to overcome writer's block is to go somewhere else. Go to a hotel room, a beach house, or to another location at the hospital or institution where you work, because then you have another environment and you have the silence and the concentration that you need to do your writing. This is efficient both for writing scientific papers, but also if you want to write a book or a novel someday. It is a very good idea to change your environment to get isolated with no internet and no disturbances, and then you can concentrate on your task.

It is important to have no distractions when writing or dictating, so if you have a smartphone, then put it on flight mode when you dictate your manuscript and also when using your computer you should not get distractions from text messages or internet-bases pop-ups. If you will use modular writing and also if you will dictate your paper on a smartphone, then preparation is extremely important. It is probably the most important part of the writing process. We use a technique called "manuscript mapping" which is a very detailed outline produced in a special way and I will cover that in a later chapter.

When you are dictating your manuscript it is important not to look back. You have to stay on track in order not to disturb your flow of thoughts and the language production in your brain. This is why we recommend you not to rewind on the recording devise and if you say something crazy then simply go to a new line and start all over again. Then in the revision phase, you will clear out all these mistakes and the final product will be readable and with easy language. You have to skip the idea of a perfect first draft because this will only create nervousness for you as a writer and this is not productive. Just go ahead and speak your manuscript according to your detailed outline and then you will be surprised to see how almost perfect your first draft will actually become. You have to use simple language and avoid overly complicated scientific words. Of course you have to use the language specifically for your research area but do not produce complicated sentences just to show-off and tell the world that you are a clever researcher. This is absolutely not necessary and will only produce text that is difficult to read. In time that will make you lose readers and this is not the purpose of writing scientific article.

    For inspiration, I would advise you to read a paper we made some years ago (dictated of course). The paper is published in The Danish Medical Journal as an open access article (in English) so you can find it at the journal website www.danmedj.dk, and the exact link to the pdf version of the article is: http://ugeskriftet.dk/files/scientific_article_files/2018-12/a4593.pdf. The citation is Dan Med J 2013;60(3):A4593. I have included the title page here but you may go to the journal link for a free full text copy of the article.

Mind-to-paper is an effective method for scientific writing

Jacob Rosenberg, Jakob Burcharth, Hans Christian Pommergaard & Anne Kjærgaard Danielsen

ABSTRACT
INTRODUCTION: The problem of initiating the writing process is a well-known phenomenon, especially for young and inexperienced scientists. The purpose of this paper is to present an effective method to overcome this problem and increase writing efficiency among inexperienced scientists.
MATERIAL AND METHODS: Twelve young scientists within the medical/surgical fields were introduced to the mind-to-paper concept. The first and last article drafts produced by each of the scientists were scored for language complexity (LIX number, Flesch Reading Ease Scale and Gunning Fog),

speed of talking resembles the speed of thinking more closely than the speed of typing text on a computer or writing by hand. Furthermore, the quality of the text is not only associated with fluency of the speech, as it is imperative that the author has relatively much knowledge about the topic [4].

The aim of the present study was to explore and describe the mind-to-paper (MTP) concept for academic writing with the use of a structured manuscript outline, dictation of the first manuscript draft and a structured learning environment. We also wanted to evaluate if a

ORIGINAL ARTICLE

Department of Surgery, Herlev Hospital

To summarize about the environment I would say: Be sure to have no disturbances. I think it is very important to go somewhere else. If you stay in your normal office environment or at home then there will always be some kind of distractions - not always external distractions but you may yourself be distracted by the fact that you are close to your normal daily tasks. Therefore, it is very good idea to go to a totally different environment, e.g. a beach house or a hotel or somewhere else and then you can do your writing or dictation of your paper. In my research group we leave our normal environment three times per year and go to beach houses and hotels and every time all participants dictate at least one scientific paper.

When you use a smartphone and talk your paper instead of writing yourself, it will ensure that your language is not too complicated because you can simply not speak very complicated sentences. You cannot speak sentences with long words or many sentences between full stops. This will make it easier to read and the end result will be very good.

When you are writing or dictating, try not to look back – try not to stop during the process and correct your words or your sentences, because you can do that in the revision phase afterwards. So do not look back and do not have the idea that you should make a perfect first draft, because that is of course nonsense. A first draft is a draft. It needs revision, so simply just write, write, write or dictate, dictate, dictate as fast as you can and do not look back. In the revision phase you can fine-tune your language and your sentences and thereby make it even better. You have to write in a simple language and this is also done more effectively when dictating your paper compared with when you are writing it yourself. If you want to use modular writing you should start with the easy parts and that is most typically the title page and the method section, but it is up to you whatever you feel is easy.

Criteria for evaluation of papers by journals

When you submit a paper to a scientific journal, then the editor will have a look at it before sending it out for external peer review. The first decision made by the editor is to judge if the target audience is correct. This means that the content of your paper will be interesting for the readers of this specific journal. An example could be if you wrote a scientific article concerning some special receptor microscopic work in an animal model and then send that scientific paper to a general clinically oriented medical journal. The readers of this general medical journal will not be interested in the laboratory work that you are presenting, so the target audience for your paper is simply wrong. You should instead send your article to a dedicated specialty journal where the readers will have more knowledge and understanding of your field of research and thereby be interested in your article. You therefore have to think this through carefully before you submit your paper to a journal.

Criteria for evaluation of papers

- **Is the target audience correct?**
- **Originality: is it new? is it a good story?**
- **Impact: an important step forward?**
- **First time publication?**
- **Can it be reproduced?**
- **Clarity: easy to follow the text?**

The next thing that the editor will consider is the originality of your research. It has to be new and it also has to be a good story for the readers. This is not to say that there is no place for replicated studies but most journals will not be happy to publish a study that replicates previous studies with exactly the same design. If you have made such a study you should not hesitate to submit your paper, but you may consider a target journal that is perhaps not the most highly ranked within this field of research.

The next thing that the editor will consider is the clarity of the text. It has to be easy to follow the text for the reader, otherwise the reader will not read your paper and then eventually the paper will not be cited. Remember that journals and thereby editors are judged, and employed actually, on the increase of the journal's impact factor, so citations are always important for a biomedical journal. In this context it is obvious that the scientific article has to be clear and easy to read because otherwise the paper will less likely be cited. The study also has to be reproducible meaning that there has to be full transparency on the study design and the methods used.

why rejection?

- **difficult (or impossible) to read**
- **no clear message**
- **instructions to authors ignored!**
- **not relevant for this journal – remember the target audience!!!**
- **author does not comply with editor's directions**

Thus, a typical reason for immediate rejection will be if the target audience is not appropriate, if it is difficult or maybe even impossible to read the text, and if the study has no clear message. Another important reason for immediate rejection is when instructions to authors are ignored.

General trends in scientific publication

- Make it easy to read (and easy to write)
- Clear (end few) messages
- Use easy language, not fancy scientific
- Journalists are coming on to the stage

The general trend in scientific publications is that it has to be easy to read and this actually may make it easier for you to write the paper. It is a very good idea to have clear and few messages in your paper and to use easy language without fancy scientific jargon. This means, that if you have a study that is quite complicated with lots of different aims and secondary outcomes, then you may consider to split your data into more than one scientific publication. This is normally referred to as "salami-publication" and it has a negative reputation. However, from the editor's point of view salami-publication is not necessarily negative because it may make your scientific article easier to read and thereby more citable for other researchers. This will potentially increase the journal's impact factor. If you decide to split your data in to more than one article the slices of course should not be too thin. The important thing is the written product that has to be easy to read and still interesting to the extent that it will be cited by others. The possible salami-slicing of your data set therefore has to be considered carefully and you should of course discuss this thoroughly with your scientific adviser and make a detailed publication plan for your total data set.

As mentioned above, it is important for the reader that you as an author use easy and readable language without fancy scientific words. It also means that the structure of the sentences should be fairly simple because otherwise it will be too difficult for the reader to follow your text. You can make a little test about this yourself because sometimes when you read a scientific article with complicated sentence structure, then the result will be, that you simply have to stop and go back to read the sentence once again. If you experience this it is a simple sign that the sentence structure is too complicated. The reader has to be able to follow the easy flow of the text while reading at a quite high pace. Otherwise it is simply too complicated and the reader may leave your article and read something else. We write papers for them to be read by as large an audience as possible so it is a bad habit to structure your text in a complicated manor because you will simply loose readers. This is one of the reasons why dictation of your article rather than writing it yourself is an extremely good idea. When you dictate an article you are simply not able to speak with a very complicated sentence structure so the end result will be much more readable than if you write it yourself. When you write yourself, we tend as authors to construct difficult language with the use of long and fancy words and with several commas and perhaps also with long (too long)mdistance between the noun and the verb in the sentence structure. All these factors will make it difficult to read and that is why you should dictate your article rather than write it yourself. When you dictate your article it is a good idea to aim for "written language" and then the end result will be somewhere between written and spoken English. Nobody is able to dictate truly written language, so the end result will be readable and still not too flat spoken English.

Chapter 2:
Things to consider

Composition of an original article

Title

You have to spend time to choose the best title for your paper. The title is very important because it will catch the reader's attention. When people search on PubMed or other search machines for scientific articles within a certain research field, then the first thing that pups up is the title of the paper. This will therefore have to invite the reader inside to read the paper itself.

It is a good advice not to pose a question in the title and instead give the answer. This means that you should give the overall conclusion in a simple sentence in your manuscript title. This is a good advice that we have learned from the newspaper journalists because they always do this in order to attract readers for the articles.

It is also a good idea to include a verb in the sentence in order to make the sentence active. You should as far as possible avoid question marks, exclamation marks and other punctuations (except a colon that may be OK) in the title because this will disturb the reader and some will actually be a little annoyed and then skip your paper and go on to something else.

Title

Purpose is to catch the readers attention

- **Don't pose a question – give the answer!**
- **Include a verb**
- **No question marks etc. (? ! "" % &)**
- **No place or year (only if very important)**

Only use geographical places or year in the title if it is very important and if it is of specific importance for the study itself. In most cases it is not important at all and instead you should just give your overall conclusion in one single sentence in the title. If you want to underline the design of the study (e.g. a randomized controlled trial or systematic review and meta-analysis) then it is common to put a colon after your title statement and then give the study design after that. An example could be "Sunlight exposure will decrease development of mental depression: a randomized controlled trial".

Introduction

In this section you have to tell the reader why the study is important. It is a very good advice to avoid long introduction sections, because then you will lose the reader and this is not the purpose. So make it brief and interesting.

The best introduction sections are probably those that consist of only two paragraphs, where the first paragraph will set the clinical problem and in very short text explain the deficit in the evidence.

IMRAD

INTRODUCTION

Why is this study important?
- **Two paragraphs**
  - **Set the clinical problem, explain the deficit in the evidence**
  - **Establish your aim or hypothesis**
- **Avoid a large number of citations in the intro**
- **Long intros lose readers - make it brief**

The second paragraph will establish your aim or hypothesis so the reader knows exactly what to expect in the rest of the paper.

You should avoid a large number of citations in the introduction section. The purpose here is not to give a systematic review of the entire evidence base for your study, but only to raise an interest of the reader by explaining the deficit in the available evidence. That is why it may sometimes be a good idea to refer to reviews in the introduction section rather than detailed original studies. This, of course depends on the research question and research area.

Methods

The methods section should explain to the reader in a transparent fashion how you performed the study. This means, that the study has to be reproducible and you have to explain your study design in detail so that others can re-do your study without contacting you.

IMRAD

METHODS

How did we do it?

- **Statistics and ethics in the last paragraph**
- **Organise in chronological order**
- **If very difficult use subheadings**
- **Do not self-plagiarize**

The methods section is often organized in chronological order according to your specific study design but this is not always the case. If the study design is very difficult you may use subheadings but most often this is not necessary.

Most journals would prefer to have the statistical methods and permissions obtained mentioned in the last paragraph of the methods section, but a few journals would actually like the ethical permission statement given up-front in the first paragraph of the methods section. You therefore have to consult the author guidelines in order to put the ethical committee permissions in the correct place in the methods section.

So, the only overall rule of the methods section is that most journals would like the statistical methods and permissions given in the last paragraph of the methods section. And remember to write with transparency so that other researchers will be able to reproduce your study.

Results

The results section is actually the most important part of an original article. The results are what the readers come for. You have to tell the reader what you found, and it is a very good idea to start with the most important findings.

This is not always followed because many journals would like the results section first to describe the sample (e.g. patients or animals) and refer to at Table 1 for details regarding the demographics of the patients included in the study. This could be the first paragraph.

If you follow this structure, then after the demographics in Table one you will go to the most important findings of your study. This means that you will start by explaining the primary outcomes and refer to appropriate tables or figures for these findings. This will be paragraph two.

After the primary outcome, then you will give the secondary outcomes in the same manner. This, will therefore be paragraph three of the results section.

Unfortunately, it is common to use some degree of data reduction when producing your scientific data. Most researchers tend to be too ambitious and include too many variables when obtaining their data and there will not be room for everything in a scientific data. When you do the data reduction you should of course not reduce only the non-significant findings, but you should stick to your design by giving the primary and secondary outcomes in the article even though they may not be statistically significant.

> **IMRAD**
>
> **R**ESULTS
>
> **What** did we find?
> - **Make data-reduction**
> - **Only the most important observations in the paper**
> - **Tables and figures are used as an alternative to text – don't duplicate**

Tables and figures should be used as an alternative to text and not duplicate exactly what is given in the text. This means, that in the text you will give a narrative summary of the details that are given in tables and figures. Overall, it is a very good idea to include both tables and figures in your article because it will increase the readability of the paper.

Discussion
Traditionally, the discussion section may be the most difficult part for you to write as a novice author.

However, if you follow the six paragraph rule given here, it will be a quite easy task to write the discussion section - and do it the same way every time. Thus, it can be quite simple if you follow a strict composition and do this every time you write an original article. Always have six paragraphs in the discussion section - never five and never seven.

IMRAD

DISCUSSION
How important is this?

- **First paragraph is a short summary of the results in words**
- **Last paragraph is the conclusion**
- **Discuss the most important findings first – be critical, compare with other studies – most important is the perspectives of your findings**
- **Most discussion sections can be cut by 50%**
- **No results in this section**

The first paragraph should give a short summary of the results in a narrative fashion, meaning without any numbers or p-values. You shall simply tell the reader in plain text what you found in your study. This is a service to the reader, because many readers will jump to the first paragraph of the discussion section and read that before they read other parts of the article. It is therefore a good advice to include a short summary of the main results in a narrative fashion in the first paragraph of the result section. We call this the "basic findings" paragraph.

IMRAD

DISCUSSION

- **Include a paragraph on study strengths and limitations**
- **Don't say "in previous work by Soper et al, it was shown that"**
- **Do say "in previous work, it was shown that..." - the citation will take you to the article by Soper**
- **Tables summarizing the literature are a lot of work and marginal value (usually)**
    - mostly show what lousy evidence is available

The second paragraph should discuss your primary outcome findings. "Discuss" means that you will compare your results with results from other studies already published in the literature.

The third paragraph should discuss the secondary outcomes of your study comparing your results with what have been previously published. Depending on your study design you may have numerous secondary outcomes, but in order to keep the discussion section as short as possible it is advisable to choose only the most important findings and discuss those in this third paragraph. In practical terms this means that you will not discuss all your secondary outcomes and this is absolutely OK.

The fourth paragraph will give the strengths and limitations of your study. Some research groups only tend to give the study limitations, but why not also give the strengths of your study. You have performed a study with hopefully a great study design, so why not underline that for the reader as well. So, in the fourth paragraph you give strengths and limitations.

In the fifth paragraph it is advisable to explain the perspectives of the study for the reader. What do your findings mean to the patients of your city, country or maybe even worldwide? Explain to the reader why your findings are important and what implications they could have on patient care in the future.

> **IMRAD – one safe way**
>
> **CONCLUSION, use one of three:**
>
> - **Further work is necessary (means you have failed)**
> - **Perhaps, possible**
> - **Another mystery solved**
>
> **Better to understate than overstate**

In the sixth paragraph you give the conclusion of the study. This is one of three: 1) further work is necessary (this means that you have failed) 2) perhaps, possible or 3) another mystery solved. In the conclusion it is better to understate than overstate. It is unfortunately a rare phenomenon to see conclusions stating that the evidence is now final and you have to immediately change patient care based on the given findings of the paper. We should of course aim for that and design studies that are final in their study design and clinical implications, but in real life it is unfortunately only rarely the case.

Many journal editors feel that most discussion sections can be cut by 50% without losing the overall quality of the paper. This should be interpreted in a way that the results are the most important content of your paper and the discussion section is only a playground where you can show that you have good overview of the literature and so on. So, don't spend too much energy on the discussion section because this is actually not where the core quality of the paper lies.

If you follow the composition guide with the six distinct paragraphs, then you are on solid ground and it will make it easier for you to come through this section of your article. Always six paragraphs for an original article.

Overall
_____

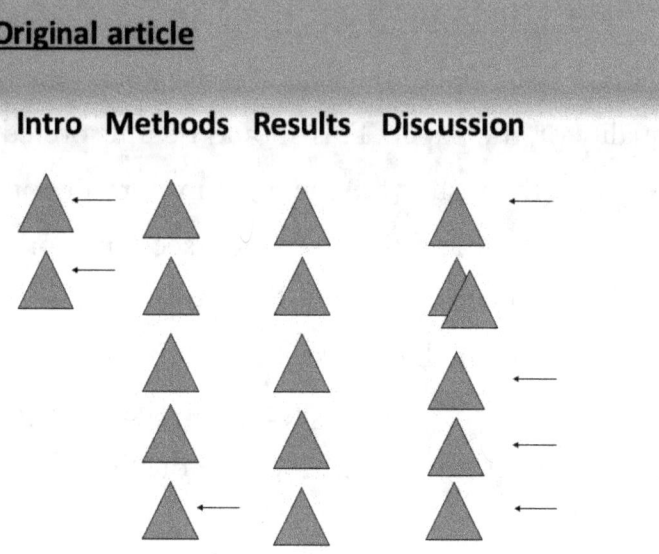

Overall, the composition of an original article will include introduction, methods, results and discussion.

The introduction section should only have two paragraphs, one giving the background of the study, and one giving the aim of the study.

The methods section could preferably be chronological in the composition and the last paragraph would most often give the statistical methods used and the permissions obtained for this study.

The results section will often start by giving the demographics of the included patients and then followed by the primary outcome findings and after that all the secondary outcome findings.

The discussion section should be composed in a strict manor using most often only six paragraphs. The first paragraph will give basic findings of the study in a narrative fashion, the second paragraph will discuss the primary outcomes, the third paragraph will discuss the secondary outcomes, the fourth paragraph will give strengths and limitations, the fifth paragraph will give the perspectives of the findings, and the sixth paragraph will be the conclusion.

Other article types

Protocol article

The protocol article has no results because it is only a publication of the study protocol. It is not, however, the protocol itself, but it has a composition of an original article without the results section.

The introduction section should preferably only have two paragraphs, the first containing the background of the study with a brief overview of the scientific evidence available, and the second paragraph would be the aim of study.

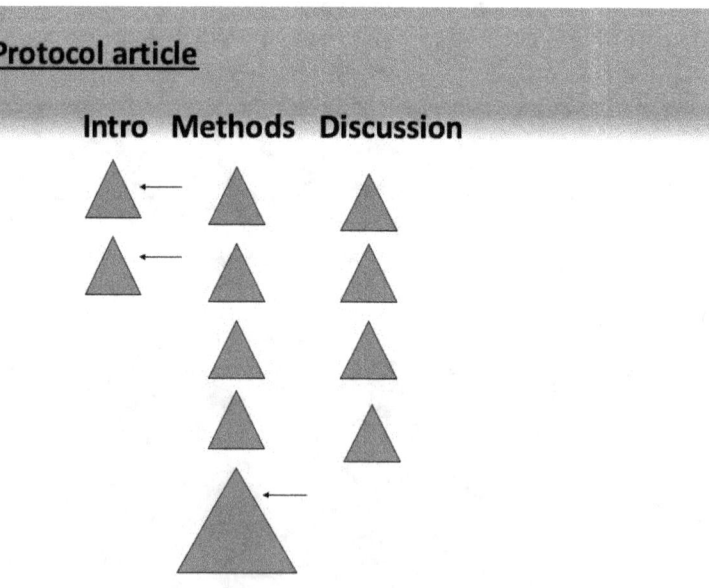

The methods section is important in a protocol article because this is where you give the reader the detailed "cookbook" of the study. In the last paragraph of the methods section it is advisable to give a detailed statistical analysis plan which is much more detailed than the statistical section in the final original article. The reason for this is that you here will define how you will perform the detailed data analysis, and this will ensure that you will not go on a "fishing expedition" when you have obtained your data.

The discussion section in a protocol article is usually quite short and will mostly discuss the possible perspectives, meaning why this study is important.

Systematic review

The systematic review is composed mostly like an original article with introduction, methods, results and discussion.

The introduction section will like in the original article only have two paragraphs: One giving the background and rationale for the study, and the second paragraph will give the aim of study.

Systematic reviews

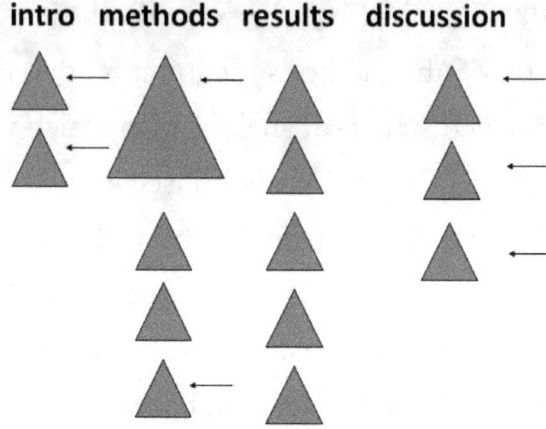

The methods section will contain details of the literature search string used to obtain the data for the systematic review. The literature search is your method for obtaining data for the review and that is why you have to give the detailed search string in order for other researchers to be able to reproduce what you have done. In the last paragraph of the methods section you may give the registration details because a systematic review can be registered at the PROSPERO website (https://www.crd.york.ac.uk/prospero/).

The results section of a systematic review will

give the most important findings first and then followed by the less important findings.

The discussion section in a systematic review is actually quite simple when you follow the PRISMA guidelines (http://www.prisma-statement.org), because when following the PRISMA guidelines you should only include three paragraphs in the discussion section for a systematic review. The first paragraph will give the basic findings, meaning that you explain for the reader in narrative terms what you have found. The second paragraph will give the study limitations, and the third paragraph will give the conclusion.

Narrative reviews

The narrative review may be a little more difficult to write because it requires that you have overview of the clinical field, and that you can see the light at the end of the tunnel. Very often, narrative reviews are therefore produced by opinion leaders or at least they have an opinion leader on board as a co-author.

The composition of a narrative review does not follow the same strict pattern as the original article and the systematic review. It is advisable to have a short introduction section with again only two paragraphs, one giving the background and one giving the one of study.

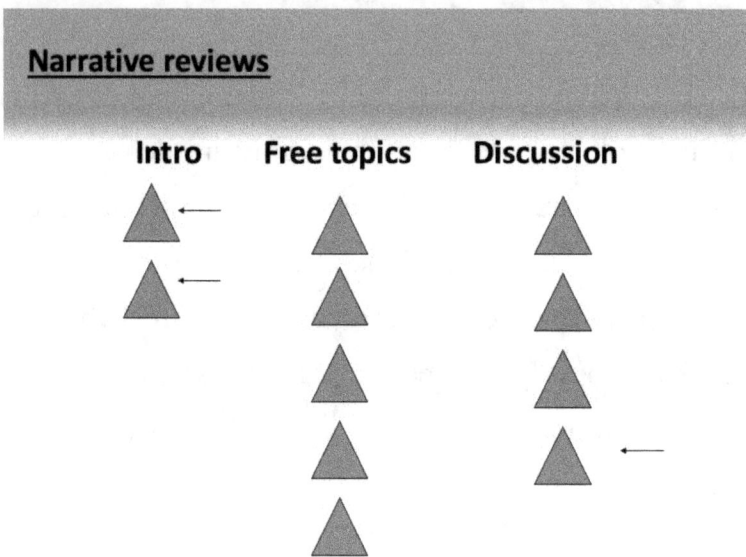

Then the narrative review typically contains a number of sections or paragraphs, which we normally would call free topics. This is where it becomes a little difficult and requires a clinical overview of the research field in order to compose these free topics in an interesting fashion for the reader.

Most reviews will also have a short discussion

section with a final conclusion at the end, but it is not a formal requirement that a narrative review has a discussion section.

Case report

A typical case report will have a short introduction section with the first paragraph giving the background and the second paragraph giving the aim.

The next section will be the case story and this is followed by a discussion section which is usually quite short.

Case reports

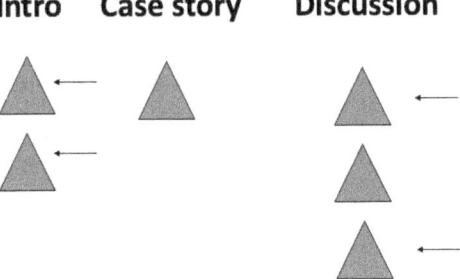

The first paragraph of the discussion section can give the summary of what this is all about and the last paragraph will of course give the conclusion. The conclusion in a case report has to focus on the learning points for the reader, because you have not produced scientific evidence like you may do in an original article or in a systematic review. The important thing to focus on in a case report is therefore the learning points and possible implications for the reader.

Editorial

An editorial is actually not a statement from the editor but most often a personal opinion from the author writing the editorial. Thus, a typical editorial is a personal statement from an opinion leader that will briefly discuss a certain area of interest and most often give strict advices to other opinion leaders, hospital administrators or even politicians. It should therefore be regarded most often as a personal statement rather than a statement from the journal itself.

There are, however, also editorials written by the editors and this is another type of editorials that will tell the reader something about journal policy etc.

Editorial

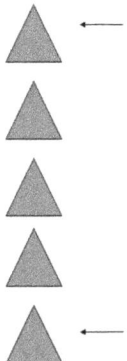

A typically editorial will be composed with an introduction paragraph and then some additional paragraphs where further details are given. At the end there will often be a quite strong conclusion with advice to hospital administrators or politicians.

Criteria for authorship

In the biomedical sciences we use the criteria for authorship defined by the International Committee of Medical Journal Editors (www.icmje.org).

> **Criteria for authorship (www.icmje.org)**
>
> **Authorship is based on substantial contributions to all these 4 criteria:**
>
> 1. [Conception and design], [acquisition of data], or [analysis and interpretation of data]
> 2. [Drafting the article] or [revising it critically]
> 3. Final approval of the version to be published
> 4. Multicenter accountability

These authorship criteria have undergone several revisions through the years, but are currently composed of four criteria, and all authors have to fulfill all those four criteria. If a person does not fulfill all four criteria, then he or she is not an author and should instead be mentioned in the acknowledgement section of the paper as a contributor. On the other hand, if a person does fulfill all the four criteria for authorship, then he or she has to be an author on the paper and this means that the name should be mentioned in the byline of the paper.

In this context it is confusing and unnecessary to use group authorship such as e.g. the "Myocardial Infarct Study Group" or something like that. It is much more transparent to simply mention all authors in the byline and all contributors in the acknowledgement section.

Some journals have limitations for the number of authors in the byline and this is a strange and unnecessary rule. If the journal wants to follow the recommendations from the ICMJE then they have to accept all authors that fulfill the four authorship criteria to be mentioned in the byline, no matter how many they are. Some studies naturally require quite a few authors and for these studies it is strange to have limitations for number of authors. On the other hand the journal of course has to secure that all authors mentioned in the byline fulfill the four authorship criteria and most journals have some kind of an authorship declaration form where the individual authors sign a statement that they fulfill all four.

The authorship criteria are given in the figure above. For authorship criterion number one, an author has to fulfill one of the three factors given in the parentheses. This means that an author should have contributed to <u>either</u> conception and design <u>or</u> acquisition of data <u>or</u> analysis and interpretation of data.

For authorship criterion number two an author has to either have drafted the article (this is typically the first author) or revised it critically (typically all the co-authors).

For authorship criterion number three, all authors have to give final approval of the version to be published. This may seem to be an easy task, but you have to get this formal, final approval from all authors. We normally send the final version by email to all authors and ask them to respond within 24 hours with a final approval. If they do not respond they are actually not authors according to the ICMJE criteria and will be removed from the author list and put into the acknowledgement section instead. If you tell this to the authors I can assure you that they will respond immediately with final approval.

The fourth authorship criterion about multi-center accountability is the newest on the list and it has produced some confusion in certain countries. This criterion does not mean that all authors have to be responsible for all details in the full scientific paper. Instead, it means that all authors should be able to point at the person who is responsible for a certain part of the paper. For instance, if you have made a study in multiple institutions or even countries you can of course not be personally responsible for e.g. some pathological evaluations of tissue made at another institution. On the contrary, you should instead be obliged to point at the person responsible for these tissue evaluations in the other institution, and thereby make it possible to clarify issues and questions regarding all aspects of the paper.

Reference management software

New researchers may ask whether they need a reference program or not. There is no clear answer to this question. Reference programs have their advantages and disadvantages and the final decision must be based on a thorough review of these.

In a reference program the researcher makes his own small database with the most frequently used references. This is typically done by automatic download from PubMed or other search engines, and then the reference program can be fed with these articles. You can of course also add references manually to the programs.

The advantage of a reference program is that it can provide references directly into a reference list in a pre-defined format, thus in the format of the specific journal that will receive your manuscript.

Another clear advantage is that if you in the writing process want to move sentences or paragraphs, then the numbering of the references will automatically be changed to the correct order. This is often very nice, since your supervisor or the other co-authors may suggest significant changes to the manuscript in the process of critical revision before submission. This is a smart feature especially if you write articles in a way that allows sentences and paragraphs to be moved in the review process within the author group. This is the so-called traditional writing technique, where your co-authors typically will see the manuscript draft for the first time when all text is written and ready for critical revision. There is an alternative way of writing papers, which is the technique that I will strongly suggest that you try, and that is to create a detailed outline or map of the paper before one single word is written on the manuscript itself. Then you can circulate this outline to the co-authors, and not until everybody has agreed fully on the outline of the paper, then you can start to write the actual manuscript. With this approach your co-authors will not need to move anything around in the revision phase, because they have already said yes to the outline, which has included the flow of paragraphs and the individual sentences with reference numbers. This specific technique will be covered in some later chapters, so I will leave it for now here. But if you use such a writing method, then the advantage of the reference program where it can automatically change numbers on your references that will not be so important anymore.

After all these positive features said about reference programs, it is very important to understand that no reference program is 100% error free. This means that when you have made your final list of references using the reference program, then you will have to turn off the coding of the references in the document, and go through your list of references manually. You will be surprised to see how many errors the program actually has made. It is often quite terrible. So never trust your reference program 100%. You have to check it manually before submission. This is very important. It means that each letter, comma, period, etc. has to be evaluated by yourself and adjusted to the final formatting. Reference programs make mistakes of various kinds, even though they obviously should not do this. One should therefore check the reference list carefully before submission, and there must not be a single microscopic error.

The reference list gives a distinct impression to the editor and the reviewers, and if there are errors in the reference list, then one might suspect that there could also be errors in the data analysis. It therefore gives a very bad overall impression, if you don't have an absolutely flawless reference list.

It may be difficult for reference software to give the correct format for example for journals who want the DOI code listed behind the article, or if the article is accepted for publication but not yet published in its final form, meaning that is has not yet received the final volume number and issue and page numbers. The only advice here is to consult the journal's reference lists and see how it is set up. Then you have to correct your own list manually to fit this specific journal style. For articles accepted for publication you will typically not indicate the term "E-pub ahead of print" which is used by for instance PubMed. In stead you will typically in a list of references in your paper just put the anticipated year of publication, a colon, and then the term "in press". However, it can vary between journals, so check out reference lists in the journal, and then you can customize your own before it is submitted.

Finally, it must be emphasized that it obviously takes some hours to become familiar with the use of a reference program. It also takes substantial time to feed it with articles and it takes again time to correct any errors in the reference list in your paper. This means that if you only have the intention to write a single or maybe a few articles, then it is a waste of time to use of a reference program. On the contrary, if you intend to produce a number of papers, and especially if they are within the same overall subject area, then it will be a good idea to select a reference program and then stick to this specific program throughout your academic career.

Problems with Internet references - web archiving is the solution

It is well known that references to pages on the Internet are not sustainable for a long time. If you use an Internet reference, it will therefore perhaps after only a few months be useless, as the provider of the website has changed the content. However, it may still be important to refer to Internet pages in scientific articles, as these may have information that is not available elsewhere. So how can we refer to an Internet page as a reference in a scientific paper and at the same time ensure that the readers of the scientific paper can actually find this information afterwards.

    There is now a clever solution to the problem. You can copy the webpage and save it forever in a web archiving solution on the Internet. There are different places to do this, and one of them is archive.org/web/. This non-profit organization offers to save copies of websites for good, and in this way ensure that when you use an Internet reference, it will always be available for the reader of your scientific article even though the owner of the website has changed the content. They have now (September 2019) saved copies of 330 billion web pages. Quite amazing I must say. Remember that this is just one of several available free service providers in this field. You simply type the link to the web page that you want to save in the "save page now" box, and then it is saved forever. It will give you a new link, that you then can include in your reference list in your scientific paper. Thus, your reference could originally look like this:

http://www.nejm.org/doi/full/10.1056/NEJMimc1411912

And after saving, the new link will look like this:

https://web.archive.org/save/_embed/http://www.nejm.org/doi/full/10.1056/NEJMimc1411912

In your scientific paper you will give the reference in the reference list followed by a web link, and in stead of giving the original weblink you will give the new weblink to the same page but saved forever in a web archive. This will ensure that your reader will always be able to find the information at a later stage.

It is an excellent initiative that was started by a single person, and the Internet archive only works on a voluntary basis and by donations. We must therefore hope that such a service can continue to ensure funds for future operations, as this initiative actually solves the problem with the use of internet references in scientific articles.

Chapter 3:
Manuscript-map

General preparations

The first thing you should consider when preparing your scientific article is to clearly define the message for the reader. It has to be simple so it will be easier for you to write the paper and it will be much easier for the reader to follow the text and get the message across.

Before preparing it further it would be a good idea if you choose your target journal because this will in some cases define details of your outline according to the guidelines for authors for that specific journal. When choosing a journal you have to be realistic and yet ambitious. Of course all papers cannot be published in the New England Journal of Medicine, but it is no crime to aim a little high, but still of course to be realistic and to choose a journal with the appropriate target audience.

How to write an original article preparations

- What is the message for the reader?
  - KEEP IT SIMPLE !!!
- Which journal are you aiming for?
  - Be realistic and yet ambitious
- Find instructions for authors and read carefully
- Make data analysis, statistical tests, tables and figures
- Organise the ideas; brainstorm – takes time!
- Find literature, read, and sort references according to IMRAD – make piles to each paragraph in the discussion-section
- Make reference list
- Detailed manuscript outline

The next step will be to find the instructions for authors and read them carefully. You have to follow the instructions for authors meticulously. It is not time for you to invent the wheel and compose your article in the way you prefer if the instructions for authors tell you otherwise.

You will have to make all data analyses, all statistical tests and produce all tables and figures to be used in the article. This has to be finalized before you dictate your article. When you have all your data available including tests and tables and figures, then you can more easily define the angle of the paper and the composition will be easier to produce.

The next phase normally is to organize the ideas in a brain-storming phase. This can be performed simultaneously with the data analysis, but it is important to consider that the brain-storming phase actually takes some time.

Coherent with this you will find the necessary literature in formal literature searches on e.g. PubMed. You will read the literature and choose the references that you want to use in your paper. These references should already at this stage be put into a formal reference list that contains numbers. The reason for using numbers is that the Dragon transcription software has a hard time recognizing author names and page numbers etc. so it is much easier when dictating the article if you dictate article numbers in parentheses instead of dictating the author names when using references that you want to include in your final article.

I would recommend that you print these references on paper instead of only having them electronically. This will make the dictation process much easier. Actually, every single text paragraph in the article should have its own set of references so you can take one pile of references and put them on the table when you dictate this specific paragraph. This also means that if you want to use the same reference both in the introduction section and the discussion section, then it is advisable to actually make two printouts of this specific reference.

When you use fixed reference numbers in the preparation phase, it will most often mean that the numbering of the references has to be changed in the end, but this is an easy task when you have your full draft of your article.

The next step which is probably the most important step of them all is to work on your detailed manuscript outline, the so-called manuscript-map (see next chapter).

When your manuscript-map is finished and you have all your references sorted in plastic folders with one pocket for each text paragraph in the final article, then you are ready to dictate the first draft of the full article in one single session.

When dictating it is advisable not to look back which means that you should never rewind on the recorder/smartphone. Simply dictate, dictate, and dictate as fast as you can. If you say something wrong then simply dictate "new line" and say it all over again, and then in the revision phase you will fix these mistakes and produce a readable first draft of your full article.

It is important to use only one day for the total dictation phase in order to keep your mind focused on this task. When using this technique you actually only have to use the references this once and when finishing the first draft you can in most cases actually skip the references and only keep the reference list.

When dictating it is important to avoid unreadable scientific language and this is best done by dictating rather than writing yourself.

Dictation technique "write write write"

- *Write first draft of the full article in one single shot!*
- *Don't look back – "write write write" - never rewind*
- *Use only one day!*
- *References only on the table this once!*

Writing style
  Short sentences, use simple words
  Avoid unreadable "scientific" language
  Use a smartphone!

You should use short sentences and simple words and this is automatically fulfilled when you dictate rather than write it yourself. When dictating you should in your mind aim for written scientific language knowing that this an impossible task. The end-product will therefore be somewhere between spoken and written English and thereby will have a nice flow throughout the text with an appropriate level of complexity of the language.

You can use an old-fashion dictaphone or any recording device that you have, but it is advisable to use a smartphone with a dedicated dictation app and then have it transcribed automatically with commercially available voice recognition software (see specific chapter about this).

The next phase will be the revision phase. The first revision will be performed only by you so you are the only one that will see all your small errors that you made when dictating. You will fix all these small mistakes and correct spelling and typing errors and maybe work on some of the weak paragraphs of your article. Typically, the title page, tables, figures, acknowledgements section, copyright statements etc. are not dictated, and in this revision phase it is normal to work on these sections as well. Cover letter and abstract should be dictated while you are in the flow phase of dictating the article.

Finally, you will make sure that references in the reference list are written strictly according to the instructions for authors and that the numbering is correct.

When you have revised your manuscript and cleared typing errors etc. then it is time to involve your co-authors once again. The involvement of co-authors should already have taken place in the manuscript outline phase (the manuscript-map) because then you have decided the angle of the discussion and the conclusions with the entire author group before you dictate your first draft. This is a great advantage, because then you will not risk that some of your co-authors will suddenly get an idea to change the angle of the paper at this very late stage. So, involve your co-authors as early as possible - already in the outline-phase - and then they will accept your angle of the manuscript before it is dictated. After the first revision that is only performed by you alone, the manuscript will now go out to all the co-authors and you will get critical feedback from all of them. If they do not give you critical feed-back they actually do not fulfill the second ICMJE authorship criterion and thereby they will actually not become authors of the paper. It is therefore important that all co-authors give critical feedback in this revision phase.

When getting feed-back from your co-authors you normally will accept all the co-author corrections. However, if they are contradictory you decide as first author what to correct. This may be a process that will take some time and may require several revision-rounds, especially with your supervisor.

When the manuscript is finished then you will send it once again to the co-authors and ask for final approval. When you have the final approval for submission you can submit your paper to an appropriate journal.

Manuscript-map

A manuscript-map is a detailed outline of all the paragraphs in the final article including references. This means, that every paragraph will have its own bullet in your manuscript-map and you will write key-words for the content of that specific paragraph and include reference numbers for the different statements that you want to include in your paragraph. These reference numbers of course will refer to the reference numbers in your reference list that you have already prepared.

Manuscript mapping

- **Detailed outline of all paragraphs including references**
- **Ongoing revision up to dictation – a working document**
- **Overview of content and message**
- **Clarification of angle with author group**
- **Move work load from writing phase to preparation phase**

The production of the manuscript-map certainly takes time and very often it may take perhaps 1-2 months of work (not full time). It is a working document that will undergo multiple revisions up to the actual dictation of the manuscript first draft.

It is important in this manuscript-mapping-phase to include all your co-authors because then you can clarify the angle of the paper with the author group before you dictate the first draft. This will often save you quite some time depending on how your co-authors, maybe especially your supervisor, will normally work with a manuscript draft.

I am pretty sure that the work-load that you now put into producing a detailed manuscript-map will not in itself constitute less working hours compared to the "old-fashioned" technique, where people typically start to write and then spend a lot of time in the writing as well as the revision phases. When producing a detailed manuscript-map you will move your workload from the writing phase to the preparation phase and it is much more rewarding for you as a writer to produce a more finished first draft compared to the "old-fashioned" technique.

Outline – manuscript map

- **Same structure as final article (IMRAD)**
- **One bullet for one final text paragraph**
- **Use words or very short sentences**
- **include numbered references**

The manuscript-map will have the same structure as the final article including introduction, methods, results and discussion sections. There should be one bullet for each final text paragraph and at these bullets you will write words and maybe very short sentences but not full sentences, because then you are writing the paper already. You have to speak your paper in order to produce a better sentence structure and a better level of language complexity compared with when you write it yourself.

When you put key-words or short sentences at these bullets it is important to include the numbered references for each sentence that you are going to produce. Then it will make your work much easier in the revision phase because you have already now decided where you will use the different references in your final article.

Before you start

- **Find and read necessary literature**
- **Make numbered reference list – OK to have too many references at this stage**
- **All results analysed with final tables, graphs, citations, statistics etc.**
- **Discuss angle with supervisor (co-authors will kick in later in the process)**
- **Decide target journal and read instructions to authors**

Before starting you will have to find and read the necessary literature. You should make a numbered reference list and it is of course OK to have too many references at this stage because you can always delete some after you have produced your first manuscript draft. All research data should be analyzed with the final tables, figures, citations (for qualitative research), statistical tests etc.

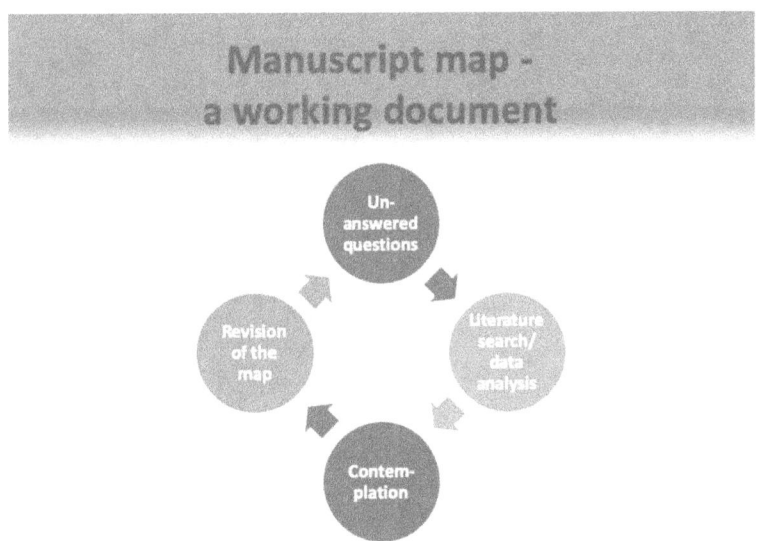

You should discuss the angle with your co-authors and especially with your supervisor in order to work in the correct direction. It is also a very good idea to decide the target journal at this early stage and read the instructions for authors, because then you will compose your article according to these author guidelines from the beginning.

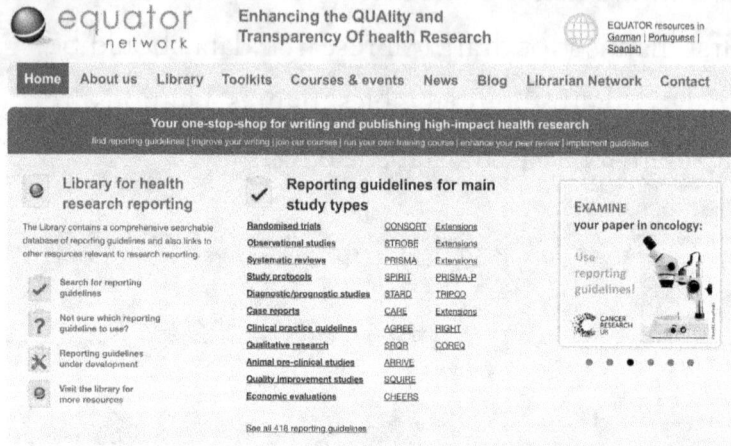

When deciding on the article composition it is a very good idea to go to www.equator-network.org and see if there is a reporting guideline for your specific study type. There are more than 400 reporting guidelines published and these guidelines are made to help you in the writing process so it is certainly advisable to go to the equator website and see if you can get help from one of these guidelines. If you find a suitable guideline you should follow it as far as possible and you should write in the manuscript itself and in the cover letter to the editor, that you have written your paper according to this specific guideline. These guidelines are made to increase the quality of the reporting of research findings so it is a good idea to follow them if possible.

Outline an original article

Introduction
- Background
- Hypothesis & aim

Methods
- Paragraph 1
- Paragraph 2
- Paragraph 3
- Ethics & statistics

Results
- Demographics (Table 1)

- Primary outcome
- Secondary outcomes

Discussion
- Basic findings
- Primary outcome
- Secondary outcome
- Strengths & limitations
- Perspectives
- Conclusion

You will compose your manuscript-map with the different sections and bullets according to the article composition given in another chapter in this book. For an original article it will typically be two paragraphs (two bullets) in the introduction section and six paragraphs (bullets) in the discussion section. Accordingly, the other article types have their own recommended compositions and they should of course be followed strictly in order to make the writing process easier and in fact also make it easier for the reader afterwards.

> **Manuscript map - a working document**
> - **Involve co-authors**
> - **Typically 2-3 times during a one-month preparation phase**
> - **Explain that it is <u>not</u> a manuscript**
> - **Ask them to comment on angle, data interpretation, structure and conclusion**
> - **No detailed corrections of language etc.**
> - **Overall acceptance from all before dictation**

It is important to stress that the manuscript-map is a working document that will take a long time to finish. You should involve all your co-authors in this process but you have to explain to them that this is not a manuscript so they will not correct spelling and grammar but only look at the overall composition and especially the angle of the manuscript.

The co-authors will typically be involved maybe 2-3 times during a 1-2 months preparation phase. Ask these co-authors to comment on the angle, the data interpretation, the structure and especially the conclusion. You should get overall acceptance on these issues before dictation of the first draft.

The absolute final preparation will be to finalize your manuscript-map, to have the final tables and figures, and to have all your references printed and numbered and in plastic pockets with one pocket for each bullet (paragraph) in your manuscript-map. When all this is available you are now ready to dictate your first draft.

Below you can see an example of a process developing a manuscript-map for a paper about reoperation rates after femoral hernia repair. The example covers the development of the introduction section for the final original article.

Overview

Introduction
- **Background**
- **Gap in the literature, lack of RCTs, ref. Cochrane**
- **Previous analysis on femoral hernia in the database... reference list**
- **This study**

- **The aim of this study was to investigate re-operation rates after femoral hernia**

The authors worked on the initial outline given in the figure above aiming at two final paragraphs in the introduction section: One giving background and one giving the aim of study. When starting the manuscript-map it is normal to write too much. Too many notes and key-word, and maybe also short sentences (see below). This stage will then evolve during several revision phases, both by yourself, and also with the co-authors. In the figures below, you can see how the different stages developed, and then the final manuscript version. It is of interest, that reference numbers are used already in the early stages, and that they go through to the final version.

Introduction
- Background.
- Femoral hernia: rare condition 2-4 % of groin hernias.
- More often affecting woman than men.
- Many different approaches for femoral hernia repair (1–4).
- Gap in the literature.
- relative few studies, and a lack of RCT, Cochrane(5).
- Register studies represents an alternative to RCT.
    - Swedish hernia register, 588 (206 emergency) femoral repairs (6), 2924 femoral hernias as a subgroup (7), 2524 elective and 1409 emergent femoral hernias (8). DHDB 1055 femoral repairs, subgroup (9). Shouldice hospital 2105 femoral repairs (10).
- This study.
- To our knowledge this is the largest cohort of femoral hernia patients published (n=5064).
- Description of DHDB (nationwide, >148.000 operations, surgical practice – not specialized center).
- First publication focusing solely on reoperation rates following femoral hernias from DHDB.
- Aim.
- The aim of this study is to investigate re-operationrates after femoral hernia and find out which method gives the lowest re-operation rate.

After multiple revisions

Introduction
- Background.
    - 10.000 repairs annually in DK
    - Femoral hernia: rare condition 2-4 % of groin hernias (1,2).
    - Often emergencies (3,4)
    - Many different approaches for femoral hernia repair (5–8).
- Gap in the literature.
    - relative few studies, and a lack of RCT, Cochrane(9).
    - Register studies represents an alternative to RCT (1).
    - Guidelines recommendation (10, 11).
- This study.
    - To our knowledge this is the largest cohort of femoral hernia patients published (n=5064).
    - Description of DHDB (nationwide, >148.000 operations, surgical practice – not specialized center).
    - First publication focusing solely on reoperation rates following femoral hernias from DHDB.
    - Aim.
    - The aim of this study is to investigate re-operationrates after femoral hernia.
    - Reoperation as a surrogate measure for recurrence.

Final article

In Denmark, approximately 10 000 groin hernias are repaired annually. Of these, 2% to 4% are femoral hernias.[1,2] Femoral hernias may pose a special risk for the patient because they often present as emergencies with suspected intestinal obstruction.[3,4] Several methods for repair of femoral hernias are used including sutured repair and different types of mesh repair with either open or laparoscopic techniques.[5-8] The fact that many approaches are currently in use reflects a rather low level of evidence for the best method of repair. Randomized clinical trials are lacking.[9] Large, prospective cohort studies are an alternative way of acquiring improved evidence regarding the best type of repair.[1] Currently, Danish[10] and European[11] guidelines for hernia repair recommend that a laparoscopic approach should be used for femoral hernia repair.

The Danish Hernia Database has prospectively recorded hernia repairs for the past 15 years and has national coverage. The aim of the present study was to investigate the reoperation rate after laparoscopic and open repair of a femoral hernia on a nationwide basis.

Exercise

Try to make a simple manuscript-map only including the introduction section of an original article. You can choose your subject yourself. It can be anything and also a purely hypothetical subject.

The introduction section should only include two paragraphs with the first paragraph giving the background of the research area and thereby explaining the lack of evidence, and the second paragraph will give the aim of study.

You should preferably only include maybe 3-4 references in the first paragraph of the introduction section. This will most often be enough.

In the manuscript-map you will then have two bullets and remember only to write single words or at the most you can give short sentences. Do not write the full sentences because then you have written the paper already.

Chapter 4:
Prepare for dictation

Required equipment

You have to have a recording device (e.g. a smartphone), software that can produce the sound file (e.g. a dictation app for a smartphone), and then some kind of voice recognition software to transcribe your sound file. You can skip the voice recognition software if you have a secretary to transcribe your dictated sound file or if you transcribe it yourself.

Required "equipment"

- iPhone, iPad, iPod touch, or Android smartphone
- Dictate + Connect (app – 17$)
- Dragon NaturallySpeaking (PC/Mac software), secretary or yourself

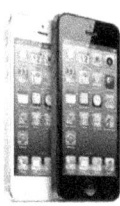 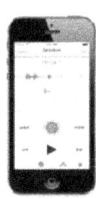 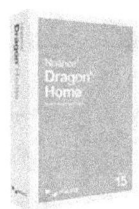 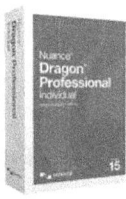

You need a recording device, and this is nowadays easy with a smartphone. It can be either an iPhone or an Android smartphone because there is the necessary software available (apps) for all types of smartphones. You can also use an iPad or even an iPod Touch because the apps available for the iPhone can also work on iPads and iPod Touch. You may of course also use the older dictaphones with tapes but then you cannot get the benefit of automatic transcription afterwards because this will need a digital sound file.

Dictate + Connect

- **Buy in iTunes or Google Play**
- **Free version available:**
  - Only 30 sec recordings
  - Only 5 recordings at the same time
- **Full version:**
  - Up to 24h in each recording
  - Unlimited number of recordings
- **Does not crash!!**

If you use a smartphone you will need to have a special app that will record your dictation. There are already various dictation apps included when you by a smartphone and there are also may free apps available to download. However, they do not seem to be stable enough to hold these sometimes quite big files that you produce when you dictate a full scientific article. We have tested a number of different apps and many of them unfortunately have problems. Therefore, we have chosen a specific app that is always stable and it does not crash during the dictation. It also gives you the liberty of producing different types of sound files and with different export options. The app is called Dictate + Connect and is available both in iTunes and Google Play. There is a free version available but it can only hold 30 seconds recordings and only five recordings at the same time. This is therefore not usable for you and you have to go for the full version if you want to use this app for dictation.

The full version of Dictate + Connect costs about 17 US-dollars and it will be possible to make sound-files up to 24 hours in each recording and with an unlimited number of recordings. The interphase is like an old-fashioned dictaphone so it is easy to start and stop and so on while recording. Most importantly it does not crash. I should say that I do not hold stocks in this company and do not have any financial interests whatsoever (maybe I wish I had), but I can fully recommend this app for dictating scientific articles.

Dragon NaturallySpeaking

- **Home (30$)**
  - Only one input device
  - Does not support Bluetooth devices
  - Does not work with Excel or Powerpoint

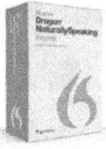

- **Premium (69$)**
  - Multiple input devices incl. email transfer
  - Multiple profiles
  - Various additional features

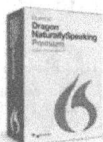

For voice recognition, meaning the software that you need to have your sound-file transcribed to a word-file, then there are also different options available out there. We have tried a few and have chosen Dragon NaturallySpeaking. This software is available at the company's own website and also for download or as a physical copy from the Amazon marketplace and of course also from many other places on the Internet.

There is a home version and a premium version and if you are going to use this regularly then you may go for the premium version. The home version currently costs 150 US$ and the premium version costs currently 300 US$ in the newest versions (version 15) on the Amazon.com website. If you go for the older version 13, then the prices are much lower (30$ and 69$). The main advantages with the new version are, that you do not have to train it and prepare it before you use it, and the error rate should be remarkably lower.

New versions available

- **No training is required!**
  - Integration with Microsoft Word
- **Home (150$)**
  - Only direct dictation to computer
- **Premium (293$)**
  - Multiple input devices incl. email transfer
  - Multiple profiles

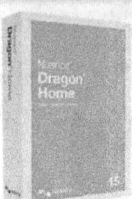
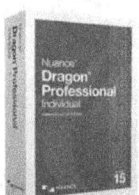

The home version can only work with one input device and it does not support bluetooth devices. Furthermore, it does not work with Excel or PowerPoint but for the purpose of dictating scientific articles you only need it to produce the text on the screen, so this is not a problem with the home version. The main problem with the home version is, that you can only use one input device and in practical terms it means that you will have to dictate your article using for instance a USB-microphone directly attached to your computer. On the other hand, when using the premium version, you can have multiple input devices including email transfer of the sound-recordings. This is very interesting because when you dictate your manuscript on a smartphone you are not bound to sit down beside your own computer when dictating the paper. This gives you freedom to dictate your manuscript anywhere you want, in a hotel room, in a beach house, or wherever you are at the moment where you get the inspiration to produce your manuscript.

After dictating on your smartphone you can download the recording either to your USB-stick or you can even email it to the computer that contains the transcription software. The premium version will also give you the opportunity to create multiple profiles and it has various additional features as well. This means that if you want to use the Dragon software on a regular basis and want the freedom to make recordings on your smartphone, then it is strongly advisable to go for the premium version instead of the home version.

There may certainly be other options available that may work just as good as the mentioned app and voice recognition software, but the equipment and software that I have chosen to highlight in this book is the ones that works for me and my research group so you can regard it as a "one safe way" to produce scientific articles by dictation. If you find pleasure and quality using other technical devices or other types of software then it is absolutely alright of course, as long as you use the dictation technique, because this in itself will clear writer's block and ensure a good final quality of your scientific article.

How to prepare equipment and software

If you have chosen to use the Dictate + Connect app (available for both iPhone and Android) then you should go to the settings and ensure that the recording quality is set to "high", the microphone's sensitivity is set to "100%" and the export audio format is "WAV". The sharing option should be chosen as "export". This will make it possible to export your recorded sound file and then have it transcribed using the Dragon NaturallySpeaking software afterwards.

Dictation settings

- **Dictate + Connect (iPhone/Andriod)**
- **Recording quality = high**
- **Microphone sensitivity = 100%**
- **Sharing as export**
- **Export audio format = WAV**

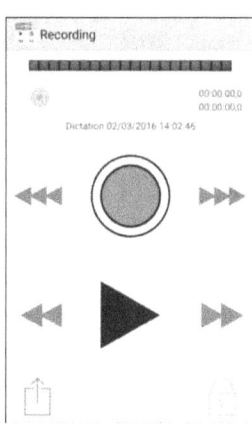

Preparation of Dragon depends on the software version. The new version 15 does not need to be trained, which is of course an advantage. The following description therefore applies to older versions of the Dragon software.

If you use a Dragon version older than the current version 15, then it is advisable to train and set up the software before you have your sound file transcribed. This can be done at any stage during the process and you can easily dictate your paper before actually preparing the software for transcription of the recorded file. In the preparation of Dragon you will have to produce a personal profile so that the program will know your accent and also know the specific glossary of your research field. The preparation comes in three steps.

How to train your Dragon

- **Speak "Alice in Wonderland", minimum 5 minutes**
- **Feed relevant documents to your profile:**
    - articles/protocols written by you, <u>Word-file</u>
    - intro/methods/discussion sections from 5-10 articles within the field, as a single <u>Word-file</u>
- **Teach Dragon during corrections**

1. You will read some pre-defined text that is available in the software. It could be e.g. "Alice in Wonderland" where you have to speak the text for a minimum of five minutes. This specific sound file will then be fed in to the system for transcription during the set up process.

2. Then you should feed relevant documents into your profile for the software to get used to the specific glossary of your research field. You can choose articles or protocols written by yourself or you can download other articles from journals and feed those into the software. You should simply copy the relevant text sections from these articles

and protocols and put everything into a single Word file. It does not matter how the text is set up because the Dragon software will read every single word and try to get used to it. This means that you should choose preferably the introduction, methods and discussion sections from 5-10 articles within the field of research and put everything in a single Word file.

3. Another way to teach Dragon your research field and how you pronounce the words, is that you use the special training option during correction of errors after the text is transcribed. It is very easy to do this with the software and it will teach the software how you pronounce the words and the glossary of the specific research field.

In the figure below you can see an example of how it helps to spend some time to train the software before transcribing the sound file. It shows the effect of feeding the software with documents, i.e. articles and protocols, before transcription of the sound file.

Eksamples of Dragon learning

Before documents:
- in 50 3C 57-year-old/6 mice: Anderson roses were created. In these Anderson roses varying degrees of ischemia were induced. Different number of supplying vessels was divided with bipolar corporation in order to create enzymatic leakage manifested as either assess of people. Tonight.

After documents:
- in 50 3C C57BL/6 mice: anastomoses were created. In this anastomosis varying degrees of ischemia were induced. Different number of supplying vessels was divided with bipolar coagulation in order to create anastomotic leakage manifested as either abscess or fecal peritonitis.

The corrected version:
- In 53 C57BL/6 mice colon anastomoses were created. In these anastomoses varying degrees of ischemia were induced. Different number of supplying vessels was divided with bipolar coagulation in order to create anastomotic leakage manifested as either abscess or fecal peritonitis.

There are numerous Dragon commands but for dictating a scientific article it is only necessary for you to use a few of those. The most commonly used are seen below. Personally, I quite often use "new line". If you say something wring during dictation, and trust ned this happens, then you simply say "new line", and then you say it agin in a better version. Don't rewind because then you will loose your dictation flow. Simply say "new line" and say the corrected sentence. When you get the transcript from the software afterwards, you can easily see where you made this error, and then you can correct it before the manuscript goes to co-authors for revision.

Dragon commands (there are numerous!)	
new line:	"new line"
new paragraph:	"new paragraph"
full stop:	"full stop"
comma:	"comma"
(	"open parens"
)	"close parens"
-	"hyphen"
(2).	"open parens two close parens full stop"

After you have dictated your manuscript draft on your smartphone, then you should export your recording as a WAV-file. A small file can be emailed to yourself but it is safer to use a cable and iTunes or simple copy-paste (for Android). You should then import your file on a computer containing the Dragon NaturallySpeaking software. This computer should be prepared in advance with your profile, because only then you will have a transcription that is readable and with not so many errors.

After dictation

- **Export recording as a file**
- **A small file can be emailed but safer by cable and iTunes**
- **Import file on a Dragon computer**
- **Dragon computer should be prepared in advance with your profile**

After you have taught Dragon how to interpret your pronunciation then you are ready to work on the first draft yourself.

Exercise

Now you can dictate the introduction section that you prepared with a manuscript map in a previous chapter.

Chapter 5: Dictation and revision of first draft

Dictation

You are now ready to dictate your first draft of the full scientific article. In this process it is important to follow the manuscript map point-by-point and not suddenly invent new text paragraphs at this stage.

You already have an overview of the literature because you have read the appropriate references and put their numbers into the different bullets in the manuscript map. So you don't have to read details in the references at this stage.

How to make the first full draft

- **Follow the manuscript map point-by-point**
- **Literature overview (don't read details now)**
- **Find a place with no distractions and dictate the full article draft in one work process**
- **Use a smartphone and voice recognition**

 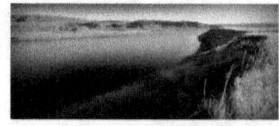

It is important to find a place with no distractions and to dictate the full article draft in one single work process. Use a smartphone and voice recognition software because this will make life easier for you. When you dictate you can use an USB-microphone if you have purchased the "home version" of the Dragon NaturallySpeaking software but if you have the premium version you can use a smartphone or an iPad and then export the recorded sound file in WAV format to be transcribed at a later stage.

- **4 paragraphs = 4 plastic pockets**

- **Every pocket contains references for that specific paragraph – no more and no less**

- **References are dictated as numbers, not names**

- **Use "new line" and "mental sticky notes"**

The references should be prepared in plastic pockets so that, if you have four paragraphs, then you should have four plastic pockets for a certain section of the article. Every pocket will contain references for that specific paragraph, no more and no less. The references are dictated as numbers, not names. This is because of the transcription software that will much easier recognize numbers than specific author names. In practical terms it means that you print all references, write numbers on them with a pen, and then make a reference list. Later on, you may have to correct the numbers slightly, but for now this reference list is the the way to go.

As mentioned in the previous chapter it is a good advice to use the term "new line" often during dictation, because you will undoubtedly say some crazy things when dictating your paper. You cannot produce a perfect first draft and you will stop the recording device numerous times during your dictation. You will probably only be able to dictate one or maybe two sentences at a time, so you have to stop the recording frequently. If you say something crazy then simply say "new line" and say it all over again.

If you suddenly get a good idea during dictation you can use so-called "mental sticky notes". This means that you will say "new line" and then make a small memo to yourself because this will also be transcribed by the Dragon software. Then after your mental sticky note, you can say "new line" again and continue with your manuscript.

Dictation – language complexity

- **Spoken versus written**
  - Aim for written scientific language
  - This is however impossible so the end result will approach spoken language and still be scientific in nature

- **Flow**
  - Mind-to-paper
  - Readability
  - Time

You should aim for written scientific language knowing that this is an impossible task. The end result will therefore be an appropriate level of language complexity somewhere between spoken and written language. The end result will approach spoken language but still be scientific in nature.

The typical scenario will be, that when you have dictated your full first draft you will probably be a little worried about the quality of the product. However, when you see the transcribed first draft it will most certainly astonish you in a positive direction because it is most often absolutely readable and at a very good quality level. Remember that you have spent a lot of time working on your manuscript-map and this has been cleared with the entire author group. You have all your data analyzed and available so the writing process itself is much easier and without writer's block. You will have a better flow through the paper, and you can certainly see that when reading your first draft yourself.

Revision of the first draft

You will be the only one to see the first transcript. This version will then be corrected for typing/spelling errors, mental sticky notes, and various weak passages, e.g. where you have used "new line" and then rephrased the sentences. These correction are fairly easy to make, and you can most probably clear everything in a few hours.

Revision - the process

- **Sentences (present/past tense, singular/plural)**
- **Paragraphs**
- **Punctuation**
- **References**
- **Figures**
- **Tables**
- **Instructions for authors**
- **Authorship and byline**

When going through your first draft you should look at all the paragraphs that typo correct (see specific chapter about this above). The punctuation should be corrected as the Dragon software will not automatically fill in "commas" and "full stops" and you may have forgotten especially to dictate commas in your sentences during your initial dictation of the first full draft. You should also work at the reference-list to ensure that the numbering is correct and that all the references are included in the reference list and the references you are not using in the paper should of course be deleted from the reference list. You should finalize all the figures and tables to their final lay-out and in this process it is of course important to follow the instructions for authors strictly.

Before sending the draft to your co-authors you should also secure the final lay-out of all figures and tables, you should make the final title page, preferably also produce the cover letter (the letter that will accompany your paper to the journal, write acknowledgements section and especially also the abstract).

Revision

- **First revision: Make ready for co-authors**
- **Other sections:**
  - **Figures and tables**
  - **Title page**
  - **Cover letter**
  - **Aknowledgements**
  - **COI**
  - **Abstract**

When everything is finished and you have such a full package of files containing the manuscript itself with the various additional files with figures etc. you are getting close to involving your co-authors. However, there are some corrections that have to be fixed before you send your masterpiece to the other authors for revision.

Many authors, especially those not having English as their first language, will have problems with present and past tense and with singular and plural. Therefore, you have to look at every single sentence in your paper and go through it critically and look for these possible errors. If your word processor (e.g. Word) has marked a word with a green or red underline it is not just to make the manuscript colorfull and entertaining for you. It actually means something, so every single word with a green or red underline should be thoroughly checked and corrected. And now, finally, it is time to involve the co-authors.

It is a good advice to write to all co-authors at once with a simple email asking who has time to go through your manuscript as the first one in the order of corrections. This is not the order of authors in the byline but simply the person who has time available for you at this stage. Then you can send the paper to this specific person and ask for critical revision. The paper then gets back to you will correct all the changes made by this specific co-author.

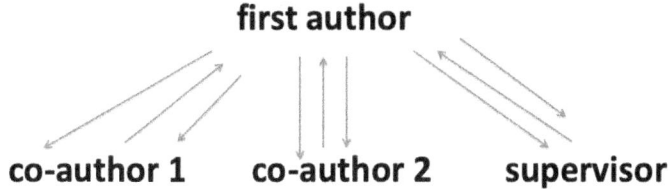

Then you send the corrected and clean version of the manuscript along to the next co-author who has indicated that he or she has time to go through your manuscript. The same process is therefore repeated and you will send the manuscript back and forth to every single co-author until everybody has given their critical revision of the manuscript. It is not a good idea to send the paper simultaneously to all co-authors, because then you will get feedback that will point in different directions. It is much easier for you as the first and co-ordinating author to get feedback from one co-author at a time and then send a "clean" corrected manuscript to the next co-author.

> **Co-authors involvement**
>
> - Criteria for authorship (www.icmje.org)
> - Get critical feedback from all co-authors
> - Revise (normally accept all co-author corrections) – if contradictory then you decide
> - Get final approval from co-authors
> - Submit

After all these corrections have been implemented in your manuscript it is time for the so-called final approval. This means that you send the final manuscript to all co-authors at once and ask them for final approval within 24 hours. If they do not give their final approval within this very short deadline, then they are actually not co-authors on the paper, because they do not fullfil the third ICMJE authorship criterion. If this happens, they will be mentioned as a contributor in the acknowledgements section instead. There may of course be situations where it is simply impossible for a person to get back to you electronically within 24 hours, but in most cases it will be possible especially if they are warned in advance that this is the working process with the paper. When you have the final approval from all the co-authors it is time to submit your article to a journal.

Chapter 6:
A few style tips

Clear paragraph typography

It is very annoying for supervisors as well as journal editors and peer reviewers to read manuscripts without a clear paragraph typography. Very often manuscripts are submitted with a quite confusing typography for the paragraphs. It should always be in the same manor, and the rules are actually quite simple.

Clear paragraph typo

First paragraph without indent
Subsequent paragraphs with indent
- No double return without indent
- No double return
- No return without indent

You can easily see how to do it if you read a newspaper article, because all the journalists have learned the correct way to do it. The first paragraph in every section of the paper should be without indent. All the subsequent paragraphs in the same article section should have a single indent. Never use double-return without indent, never use double return, and never use single return without indent. If you mix these different ways of marking the shift to a new paragraph then the reader will be quite confused and so will the journal editors and production team.

In practical terms, it means that when you start your introduction section you may have your headline "Introduction". Then you have a single return and the text will now start without indent. When you go to the next paragraph, but still in the introduction section, you will have a single return with a single indent. The same pattern should be used in all the different sections of the article (methods, results and discussion).

Delete unnecessary text

Many researchers tend to produce sentences with too many words. Therefore, when you revise your paper you should look for this and condensate the sentences to as little text as possible. An example can be seen in the figure below.

Delete unnecessary text

"This paper provides a review of the basic tenets of cancer biology study design, using as examples studies that illustrate the methodological challenges or that demonstrates succesfull solution to the difficult inherent in cancer research."

"This paper reviews cancer biology study design, using examples that illustrate specific challenges and solutions."

As you can see, the same meaning can be said in a much simpler sentence without loosing information. Another example can be seen in the next figure.

"Brain injury incidence shows two peak periods in almost all reports: rates are highest in the young people and elderly."

⬇

"Brain injury incidence peaks in the young and in the elderly."

You should therefore look at all your sentences in a critical fashion, so that they become simple and easy to read. Thereby they also become easy to understand. This is one of the main reasons why dictation of scientific articles are better than writing them yourself. It is almost impossible to dictate such difficult sentences.

Unfortunately, difficult language can bee seen in almost all journals. In the figure below you see text from a paper published in the highly estimated journal Cell.

Cell. 2011 October 14; 147(2): 370–381. doi:10.1016/j.cell.2011.09.041.

An Extensive MicroRNA-Mediated Network of RNA-RNA Interactions Regulates Established Oncogenic Pathways in Glioblastoma

"Dysregulation of physiologic microRNA (miR) activity has been shown to play an important role in tumor initiation and progression, including gliomagenesis (1-5). Therefore, molecular species that can regulate miR activity on their target RNAs, without affecting the expression of relevant mature miRs, may play equally relevant roles in cancer."

This very complicated statement can be abbreviated to the following:

"Changes in microRNA expression play a role in cancer, including glioma. Therefore, events that disrupt microRNAs from binding to their target RNAs may also promote cancer."

You can see, that if you look at your sentences with a critical view it is very often possible to abbreviate (or delete) some of the sentences and thereby produce a shorter version but still with the same message to the reader.

When working at your manuscript draft it is also a good idea to look critically on the use of acronyms. Use of acronyms will slow the reader and it is very annoying to read a paper with many acronyms. Try to use only the most well-established acronyms like CT scan or MRI and most other acronyms should simply be avoided. The reason to use acronyms is in fact often laziness from the author's side and it will certainly not help the reader.

Another important issue is to look at the distance between the subject and the verb in each sentence. The distance should preferably be short because otherwise readers may have to read the sentence more than once in order to understand the meaning.

"Therefore, molecular species that can regulate miR activity on their target RNAs, without affecting the expression of relevant mature miRs, may play equally relevant roles in cancer."

Distance between subject and verb   Acronyms will slow the reader

Avoid certain terms and fillers

Even though you have dictated your paper with the aim to go for a language level corresponding to written scientific English we all know that this is not possible so there will be some spoken jargon or slang in your paper. In the revision phase you should therefore try to avoid terms like "as it is well known ….", "it has been shown …", "it can be regarded that …", and so on.

Avoid terms like

- "As it is well known…"
- "It has been shown…"
- "It can be regarded that…"

You should also as far as possible avoid fillers like "very", "quite", "really", "basically", "generally", "extreme", and "important".

Avoid fillers like:

- "Very"
- "Quite"
- "Really"
- "Basically"
- "Generally"
- "Extreme"
- "Important"

There are some spoken terms that can be appropriately replaced with more simple words. For example "a majority of…" can be replaced with "most …", and you can see other relevant examples in the figure below. If you use software like Grammarly or similar, then these phrases will often be picked up in the revision phase.

Relevant substitutions

- **A majority of...**   most...
- **A number of...**   many...
- **Are the same opinion...**   agree...
- **Less frequently occurring...** rare...
- **All three of the...**   the three of...
- **Due to the fact that...**   because...
- **Have an effect on...**   affect...

I have a personal hobbyhorse and that is to use disease names as adjectives instead of nouns. This means that you should not call a patient with diabetes a "diabetic". This will stigmatize all patients with diabetes and assume that the diabetes is the most important or only relevant descriptive factor for the individuals. This is not OK. If a patient has diabetes and you call him a diabetic then you are signaling that diabetes is the only thing that actually characterizes this complicated and wonderful person. It is therefore negative and somewhat patronizing to use the disease names as nouns. Likewise, there are no "STEMI-patients". Instead you have patients with "STEMI". Cancer patients do not exist – instead you have patients with cancer.

Avoid name dropping

It is a bad habit to use name dropping in the running text of a scientific paper. Name dropping means that you mention the name of the author of a given reference instead of just giving the reference number in parentheses at the end of a sentence. An example could be like this: A shown by Smith and co-workers it is evident that … (ref). Instead, you should simply state: It has been shown that …. (ref).

The reason why you should avoid name dropping in a scientific paper is that it will slow down the reader. When reading a sentence including an author name the reader will automatically pause for some milliseconds and try to find out if this name is important, if he or she should know this specific author by name.

You may think that this is a small thing, but all these disturbing elements in the running text like name dropping and use of abbreviations will irritate the reader and ultimately it may cause the reader to actually leave your article and move on to read something else.

There is no reason whatsoever to use name dropping in a scientific article and you should instead simply use the reference number at the end of the sentence and thereby refer the reader to the appropriate background literature if the reader wants to know more about the subject.

There may of course be exceptions to this general rule. If an author name is a kind of an institution in the specific research area maybe naming a measurement scale then it could be justified to give the author name in the running text. However, it is advisable to try to avoid name dropping as much as possible.

Medical writing tips and tricks

This chapter will include various examples that I have picked up through the years as a scientific supervisor, as a peer reviewer, and as a journal editor. I have been a journal editor for now 16 years and served 7 years on the ICMJE so I have seen quite a lot of manuscripts in my time. The errors given in this chapter is what I have found to be of interest to give to you. The examples will be presented in a figure, and then discussed afterwards in figures and text. Let's start.

Is there a mistake here?

- **Melatonin levels were higher in men compared to women**

When you use the term "compared" it is most common in written articles to write "compared with" instead of "compared to". There is not so sharp a difference in spoken language, but "compared" with is regarded as being softer than "compared to".

compared with - compared to

- "With" more used than "to" in articles
- Not so sharp difference in spoken language
- Compared with is "softer"
- Compared with something almost the same
- Compared to something completely different

"Compared with" is often used when you compare something that is almost the same, whereas "compared to" is used when you compare something that is completely different. In scientific papers it is most common to compare something that is almost the same and not for instance to compare a ship with a house. The next example can be seen in the figure below.

Mistake?

- **Pommergaard H-C, Andresen K. Effect of Intercourse on Mood Level in Healthy Volunteers. J Mood Physiol 2014; 23: 106-8.**

The problem here is the use of capitals within title of the article in the reference list. You should never use capitals in references, also not when it is actually printed with capitals in the journal article itself. In a reference list the title words of a reference are always given with small letters.

Capitals

- Capitals in trade names but not in generic names (Panodil vs paracetamol)
- On Day 1 of Experiment 2
- As shown in Table 2 and Figure 1
- Never capitals in references, also not when it is printed like that

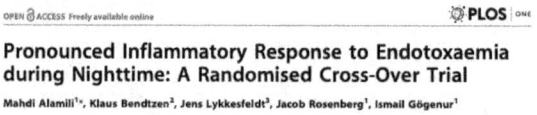

Pronounced Inflammatory Response to Endotoxaemia during Nighttime: A Randomised Cross-Over Trial

Mahdi Alamili[1]*, Klaus Bendtzen[2], Jens Lykkesfeldt[3], Jacob Rosenberg[1], Ismail Gögenur[1]

Capitals are used in trade names but not in generic names for drugs. There is a tendency now to write for instance Day 1 of Experiment 2 with capital letters, but this is to my best knowledge actually not correct written English. It is however a trend in scientific writing. The same goes for Table 2 and Figure 1 where T and F are most often written with capitals. The next example can be seen in the figure below.

Mistake?

- **Melatonin levels were higher in men. This was not expected.**

The message here is that you should always only use a single space after full stop. The exception from this rule is found in internal "full stops" in acronyms. Examples are e.g. and i.e. where there is no space after full stop. But never two spaces after full stop.

Full stop

- **Only a single space after full stop**
  - Exception in "internal" full stops in acronyms: e.g., i.e.
- **No more than one full stop if the sentence ends with an acronym with a full stop – e.g. etc.**
- **No full stop in acronyms with capitals (NATO, USA) or in routes of administration (im, iv, sc)**

Another exception is that you do not use full stop in acronyms with capitals such as NATO and USA or in routes of drug administration such as im, iv, and sc. The next example can be seen in the figure below.

Mistake?

- **Effect of sunburn on metabolism of alcohol: A systematic review.**

The message here is that you should not always use a capital latter after colon. The correct way of giving the above article title is therefore "Effect of sunburn on metabolism of alcohol: a systematic review". Information on the article or study retype is often given after a colon in the title of the paper, and in these cases we always use small letters after colon.

Colon

- **Not always a capital after colon**
  - Effect of sunburn on metabolism of alcohol: a systematic review
- **Be carefull when using colon in the running text**

Overall, I would say that you should be a little careful when using colon in the running text because it will imply sophisticated sentence structure, and this is not the goal when writing scientific papers where the text should be flowing and easy to read.

The same goes for use of semicolon that you should hopefully not use very often. The reason why should try to avoid colon as well as semicolon in the running text is that it makes the text a little harder to read. It creates breaks in the reading flow, and we don't want this. It may, of course, sometimes be appropriate to use them, but my message is just to be a little careful not to use them often.

Semicolon

- **Used to separate different things**
    - On one side it is like this; on the other side it is like this
- **When you want to indicate a longer reading pause than after a comma**
    - The committee dealing with the question of commas agreed on a final text; however, the issue of semicolons was not considered
- **Can be used as a comma-separator, if there are commas in what you want to separate**
    - $r=0.77$, $p<0.02$; $r=0.45$, $p<0.05$

A semicolon is used to separate different things (see example in the figure above). You can also use a semicolon when you want to indicate a longer reading pause than after a comma (again see example in the figure above). You may also use a semicolon as a comma separator if there are commas in what you want to separate. An example of this is when stating various results and p-values (see example above). Let's go on to another problem.

Mistake?

- **Sugar, beef, milk and butter**

When listing a number of nouns, it is often done with the inclusion of a comma before "and" at the end. Therefore, the words in the figure above would most often be stated as "sugar, beef, milk, and bitter". It is, however, OK not to include this last comma before "and" but most authors tend to do it when writing scientific papers.

For a non-native English-speaking person comma rules in English may be little difficult. In general, in English written language a comma indicates a pause. So, you can listen to the sentence when reading it aloud and then often you can actually hear where the comma should be. As a general rule written English does not use many commas, so if you are in doubt, then perhaps you should leave it out. We go on to another example.

> **Mistake?**
>
> - **Furthermore melatonin levels were higher in men compared with women**

Commas are always used after all the small "start-words" in sentences such as furthermore, moreover, however, in addition, in conclusion, etc. Thus, the sentence in the figure above should be "Furthermore, melatonin levels were higher in men compared with women".

Comma

- **Comma after alle the small "start-words" in sentences: Furthermore, Moreover, However, In addition, In conclusion,**
- **Comma before and after "however"**
  - There were three boys, however, one of them was a girl
- **Comma before and after or before "respectively"**
  - The values in group A and B were 1 and 2, respectively.
  - The values in group A and B were 1 and 2, respectively, and they all died.

There will be a comma before and after "however" when this word is used in the middle of a sentence, and the same goes for "respectively". If "respectively" is put at the end of the sentence, then we out a comma before "respectively" (see example in the figure above). Now we move on to another example.

Mistake?

- **Melatonin levels was higher in men compared with women**

The message here is the (unfortunately) very common errors with singular and plural versions of verbs and nouns. In the sentence above "was" should of course be "were" because "levels" are plural. The typical errors are was/were, has/have, is/are and s on the nouns for the plural versions. It impresses me how it can be so difficult. It is most often very simple, and Word will also help by underlining the wrong version with a green line.

Singular/plural

- **GRRRR! Why is it so difficult?**
- **Look for the green (and red) lines in Word**
- **Read ALL sentences one by one and check for**
  - was/were
  - has/have
  - is/are
  - s on the verbs

The best recommendation is to correct all green (and red) lines in Word, and very carefully read all sentences in the article and decide whether the verb should be singular or plural. Make this part of your standard revision process, and then it should be all right. Let's go on to another example.

Mistake?

- **All NSAID's are ulcerogenic**

The apostrophe is used only when giving the possessive form of nouns. Then the noun is marked by and apostrophe followed by an "s". After the plural ending (s), however, the apostrophe comes after the "s", and in singular, the apostrophe comes before the "s". If the name ends with an s then you follow the same rules, e.g. "Mr. Jones's car". You can see examples in the figure below.

Apostrophe

- **The possessive form of nouns is marked by an apostrophe followed by an –s. After the plural ending "s", however, the possessive s is omitted**
  - one month's patients
  - four months' patients
- **If the name ends with an s you follow the same rules**
  - mr. Jones's car
- **No apostrophe when used for plural of an acronym**
  - four UFOs, ten 747s, NSAIDs, RCTs

The apostrophe is not used when s is used for plural or in acronyms. Examples could be "four UFOs, ten 747s, NSAIDs, or RCTs.

The next thing I would like to discuss is the use of acronyms. In general, you should be very cautious with acronyms. The reason is that acronyms will often decrease the speed of reading, and sometimes the reader may have forgotten what the acronym meant and then has to go back and look for the definition. This is very annoying, so skip as many acronyms as possible.

Acronyms

- **Be cautious here**
- **Should make it easier for the reader – not for the author**
- **Use only standard abbreviations**
- **Write full name first time it occurs**
- **Remember that abstract, tables and figures are "independent" parts of the manuscript**

The basic reason for using an acronym should be to make it easier for the reader and not make it easier for the author. Think about this for a moment. Why do you use acronyms? To save time and energy? Are you just a lacy author? The aim is not to make it easier for the author, but easier for the reader. Therefore, you should never introduce new acronyms that are not standard in the literature. A good example is CT scan. Nobody nowadays would write "computer tomography scan" because CT is such a standard term during daily life. Therefore, CT as an OK acronym to use.

If you use acronyms, then remember that the

abstract and table and figure legends are considered to be independent parts of the manuscript so that you should write the full name also the first time you use an acronym in these specific manuscript sections. OK let's move on.

Mistake?

- **Two l of alcohol per person corresponding to 2,000 mL**

The problem here is that typically liter is abbreviated with a capital L whereas milliliter is abbreviated by small letters ml. There are some different traditions in this context and if you are in doubt you should look at previous articles published in that specific journal and then you will get a good impression of the preferred way of using these acronyms in that specific journal. You can see other relevant examples in the figure below.

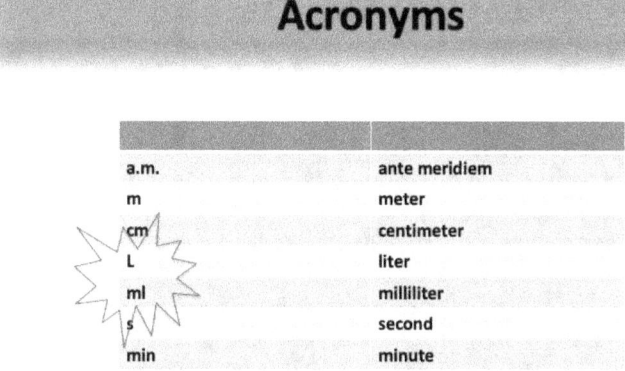

Then we move on to another problem. That is the use of spaces.

Mistake?

- **Melatonin levels were 25 % higher in men compared with women**

The problem in the figure above is that normally there is no space before % (25%). On the other hand, if you give a result like an amount of ml there is a space between the number and ml. This could be "25 ml". A space is always used in formulas' (a + b = c). When given references in parentheses there should always be a space before the open parenthesis. Thus, the correct way would be "it was shown in a previous study (1)" and not "it was shown in a previous study(1)".

Space

- **No space before % (25%)**
- **Space in results (25 ml)**
- **Space in formulas (a + b = c)**
- **Space before the reference parenthesis**
  - It was shown in a previous study (1)
  - It was shown in a previous study(1)

Of course, there are numerous other examples that may be relevant for you, but I have just chosen the ones that I most often have encountered in scientific articles.

Chapter 7:
Closing

Closing remarks

I hope that you have found the information in this book to be of value and I can assure you that if you follow these instructions you will most probably skip the most common signs of writer's block and produce a full first article draft in a single day.

Of course, you can not do all the work with an article in a single day because there is quite an extensive preparation phase with a production of a detailed manuscript-map and also a revision phase after the dictation itself. However, when structuring the different phases of the article production with a detailed manuscript-map, dictation and subsequent revision, then you will save yourself some time and negative energy and thereby hopefully increase your scientific production and also increase the quality of the written papers.

Take home messages

- **structure the process**
- **manuscript map**
- **dictation (!)**

- **one safe way**

There are of course many ways to write papers and the technique given in this book is just "one safe way" to do it with most often a very good result.

Other books in this series

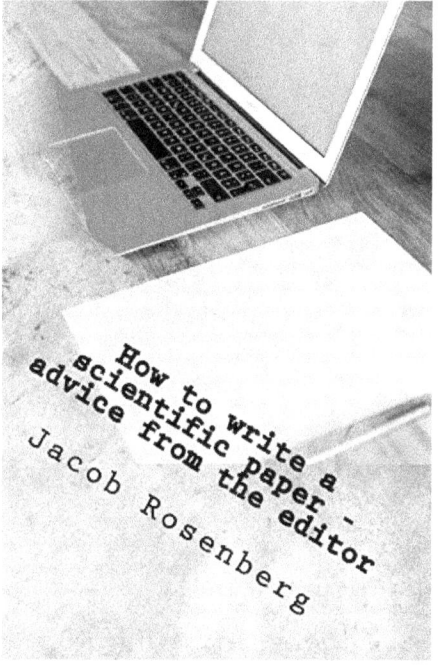

How to write a scientific paper: advice from the editor. Ultimate Researcher's Guide Series, Volume 1.

Available as paperback and kindle edition on all Amazon platforms.

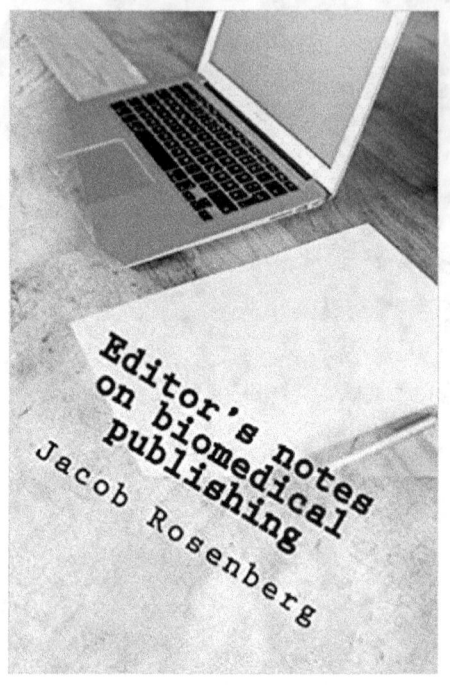

Editor's notes on biomedical publishing.
Ultimate Researcher's Guide Series, Volume 2.

Available as paperback and kindle edition on all Amazon platforms.

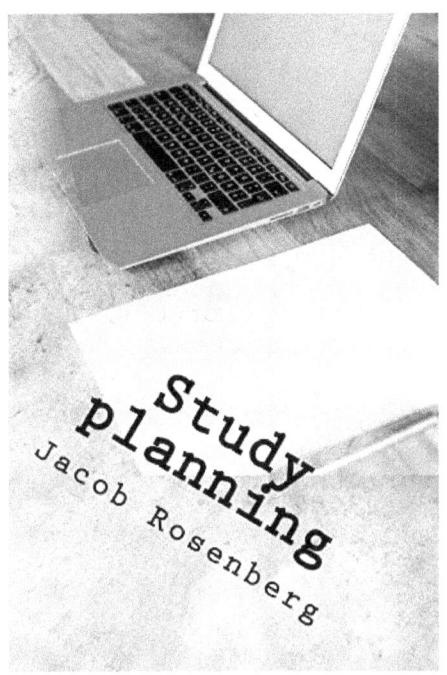

Study planning. Ultimate Researcher's Guide Series, Volume 3.

Available as paperback and kindle edition on all Amazon platforms.

About the author

Jacob Rosenberg (1964) was born and grew up in Copenhagen, Denmark. He is professor of surgery at the University of Copenhagen, and chief surgeon at the Gastro-unit, surgical section, Herlev Hospital (also in Copenhagen).

The author page at amazon.com is:
https://www.amazon.com/author/jacobrosenberg

Notes

Notes

Contact information

jacob.rosenberg@regionh.dk

www.ingramcontent.com/pod-product-compliance
Lightning Source LLC
Chambersburg PA
CBHW070638220526
45466CB00001B/215